MANFOOD

5:2 FAST DIET
MEALS FOR MEN

CookNation

MANFOOD: 5:2 FAST DIET MEALS FOR MEN

SIMPLE & DELICIOUS, FUSS FREE, FAST DAY RECIPES FOR MEN UNDER 200, 300, 400 & 500 CALORIES

Copyright © Bell & Mackenzie Publishing Limited 2014

ISBN 978-1-909855-69-4

A CIP catalogue record of this book is available from the British Library

DISCLAIMER

CONTENTS

UNDER 400 CALORIES   **61**

UNDER 500 CALORIES

EXTRAS

OTHER COOKNATION TITLES

INTRODUCTION

If you're a man and you're looking to lose weight by following the 5:2 Diet then this book is for you.

If you are reading this book you've most likely decided you're carrying a few extra pounds you want to get rid of.....or maybe someone has gifted it to you and is dropping a hint?! Whatever the reason you probably recoil at the thought of dieting but increasingly you keep hearing about the 5:2 Fast Diet and the word is IT WORKS. It's all over the news, celebrities are endorsing it and maybe even some of your friends or family are following it. So, what the hell, you've decided to give it a go and make a commitment to losing some weight. If you're a man and you're looking to lose weight by following the 5:2 Diet then this book is for you.

In it you'll find a bunch of really simple, delicious and nutritious fast day recipes all under 600 calories. Each is specifically targeted at men, balancing protein, carbs, fruit and veg. Whether you fancy yourself in the kitchen as a Michelin star chef or can't tell your penne from your paella, you'll love these MANFOOD recipes. Each serves one and most can be prepared and cooked in less than 30 minutes. Job done!

IF YOU ARE NEW TO THE 5:2 DIET HERE'S HOW IT WORKS

The principle is very simple. You eat what you like for five days of the week and limit your calorie intake for the remaining two days. On your two fast days, calories are restricted to 600 per day (500 for women – sorry girls!). You can choose your fast days each week, changing them to suit your schedule and lifestyle and they can be consecutive or apart.

What's great about the 5:2 Diet and one of the main reasons it has become so popular is its flexibility and freedom. You get to choose what to eat and when to eat; you can work your fast days around work, family, your social life and gym. The only restriction is limiting your calories for just two days a week and eating normally for the other five. Forget about committing yourself to drastic calorie deficits seven days a week and feeling miserable. The 5:2 Diet approach is a real motivator. It's got to be worth a go right?

The 5:2 Diet first hit the headlines in August 2012 following a BBC Horizon documentary called 'Eat, Fast And Live Longer' presented by doctor and journalist Michael Molesley. While the practice of fasting is not new, the TV show popularised intermittent fasting for weight loss and hailed it as revolutionary by eating what you want for most of the week and still losing weight.

On top of the weight loss benefits, research has shown that following the 5:2 Diet can reduce levels of IGF-1 (insulin-like growth factor 1, which leads to accelerated ageing), activate DNA repair genes, and reduce blood pressure, cholesterol and glucose levels as well as suggestions of a lower risk of heart disease and cancers.

So in short, the 5:2 Diet works by restricting your body to fewer calories than it uses. Most importantly is that it does this in a way that remains healthy and is balanced by eating normally for the other five days of the week. If, for whatever reason, you need to lose some pounds, then the 5:2 approach could be the best diet for you. So dive in to our MANFOOD recipes and good luck!

READ THIS! SOME THINGS YOU NEED TO KNOW

The 5:2 Fast Diet is....drumroll..... a diet! A diet meaning restricting your calorific intake in some shape or form which, let's be realistic guys, isn't always going to be easy. On your fast days you will be hungry at first, feel a little lethargic and maybe even a bit irritated and agitated (watch out friends and family!) So while this might all sound very obvious, it's good to prepare yourself so you don't fall at the first hurdle. Plan your fast days in advance. There's little point in fasting on the day you have to take business clients out for dinner or when you've arranged to go out with the boys for a night out.

Be realistic about your meal sizes

If Texan-sized meat feasts are what you are used to then get ready for some changes. 600 calories is your limit on a fast day. How you break that up is up to you. You can skip some regular mealtimes like breakfast and/or lunch and look forward to a full meal in the evening or snack healthily throughout the day. Whichever gets you through your fast day - just remember it's going to be less than you would normally eat. The good news is we've made our recipes as tasty and delicious as possible within the calorie limit and of course remember that you have 5 days of the week to eat normally.

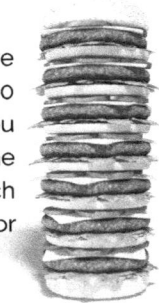

If you exercise regularly, try not to plan your fast days on the same day you train. Going to the gym when you might be feeling lethargic and hungry might not be productive.

Anyone can cook our MANFOOD recipes. They are all easy to follow – you don't need to be a magician in the kitchen. While we haven't used any 'cheat' ingredients in this book, there are some great pre-prepared ingredients that will speed up the prep time if you're in a hurry or maybe just not the type of guy who likes to spend any more time in the kitchen than is absolutely necessary. Excellent time savers include microwave rice, lazy garlic, lazy chilli, lazy ginger, cooked chicken breasts, pre-sliced onion, prepared vegetables, washed salad and low fat grated cheese. They might add to your shopping budget but they're a godsend to have in the fridge for super quick meals. Check out some essential store cupboard ingredients here to get you started.

600 Calories includes drinks! Before you plan all your fast day calories on food, remember a man needs to drink! Unless you drink nothing but water (and that's not a bad idea), beverages mean calories. If you can, stick to black teas and coffee. White coffee could be 20 calories but multiply that to 3 cups a day and you're making a serious dent in your calorie limit. No alcohol!

Get yourself two decent non-stick pans. Not only will it prevent your food from burning (less time washing up!), but any oil you use for cooking will go further. Less oil means less calories!

Snacks. No problem but they still count towards your fast day calories. Avoid them altogether unless you plan to eat little and often throughout the day on your fasting days. Snickers and crisps are obviously a no-go area!

Eat normally for 5 days...but don't go overboard. What's great about the 5:2 Diet is the flexibility to eat what you like for five days of the week while limiting your calorie intake for the remaining two. However when we say 'eat normally' we mean sensibly. The recommended daily calorie intakes for men is 2400-2500. Try not to have a blow out, gorging on unhealthy snacks, treats and fast foods. Just eat well and sensibly. The size of the portion that you put on your plate will significantly affect your weight loss efforts. Filling your plate with over-sized portions will obviously increase your calorie intake (even on your non fast days) A correct sized portion is generally the size of your clenched fist. This applies to any side dishes of vegetables and carbs too. You will be surprised at how quickly you will adopt this as the 'norm' as the weeks go by and you will begin to stop over-eating.

Get advice. If you suffer from any health issues you should first seek the advice of a health professional before embarking on any form of diet. Got it?

WHAT'S THE BEST WAY TO PLAN MEALS ON FAST DAYS?

There are a few different ways you can approach your fast days. The key is to plan ahead and think about what's going to be happening in your day and choose the best option to work with your schedule and lifestyle.

You could:
- **Skip breakfast, eat lunch & dinner.**
- **Skip lunch, eat breakfast and dinner.**
- **Eat little and often throughout the day.**
- **Eat one large meal and very little else.**

Our recipes range from 200 calories to 500 calories which means you can select meals and snacks which best suit your fast day. For example if you decide to skip breakfast you could have Sweet Chilli Salmon for lunch and Baked Lemon Chicken for dinner with 50 calories to spare for drinks.

THE BIG QUESTION...HOW MUCH WEIGHT WILL I LOSE?

Research suggests that you could lose 1 pound or more per week following the 5:2 Diet. Stack that up over a number of weeks and you could well on the way to achieving your weight loss goals as well as improving your overall health and immune system.

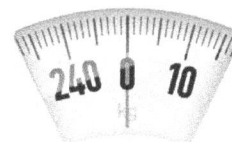

You should start seeing results by the end of your first week in most cases! Obviously everybody is different, but typically many will see a greater weight loss at the beginning, followed by a slowing down then eventually settling around a stable healthy weight.

AVOID THE PITFALLS

Let's face it, sticking to any plan needs willpower and motivation and sometimes we just mess it up. If you do, don't beat yourself up, just brush yourself down and get right back on it. Half the battle is avoiding some well known pitfalls so we're giving you a heads-up by listing some of the more frequent obstacles that can be avoided and tips for getting through your fast days and achieving your goals.

- **Slow down those jaws!** Eat. Take it slow. There's no rush. Feeding like a ravenous animal is no good for your digestive system and chances are you'll be looking for second helpings before your body has even had the chance to feel satisfied.

- **Chew.** It sounds obvious but you should properly chew your food and swallow only when it's broken down and you have enjoyed what you have tasted.

- **Wait.** Before reaching for second helpings wait 5-10 minutes and let your body tell you whether you are still hungry. More often than not, the answer will be no and you will be satisfied with the meal you have had. A glass of water before each meal will help you with any cravings for more. Remember you are on a fast day and restricting your calories. Be realistic about what to expect.

- **Avoid too much exercise on your fasting days.** Eating less is likely to make you feel a little weaker, certainly to start with, so don't put the pressure on yourself to work out.

- **Avoid alcohol on your fasting days.** Not only is alcohol packed with calories (and by the way that includes light beers), it could also have a greater effect on you than usual as you haven't eaten as much so lay off the booze boys.

- **Don't give up!** Even if you find your fasting days tough to start with, stick with it. Remember you can eat what you like tomorrow without having to feel guilty.

- **Drink plenty of water throughout the day.** Water is the best friend you have on your fasting days. It's good for you, has zero calories, and will fill you up & help stop you feeling hungry.

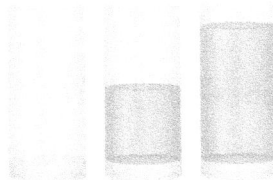

Have a glass before and also with your meal. No brainer.

- **When you are eating each meal, put your fork down between bites** – it will make you eat more slowly and you'll feel fuller on less food.

- **Brush your teeth** immediately after your meal to discourage yourself from eating more.

- **Have clear motivations.** Think about what you are trying to achieve and stick with it. Keep your eye on the prize. Remember you can eat what you want tomorrow.

- **If you get food cravings** (and you will), acknowledge them, and then distract yourself. Go out for a walk, phone a friend, play with the kids, or annihilate something on the PS3!

- **Whenever hunger hits**, try waiting 15 minutes and ride out the cravings. You'll find they pass and you can move on with your day.

- **Remember - feeling hungry is not a bad thing.** The norm is to snack on the smallest hunger pangs - we've forgotten what it's like to feel genuinely hungry. Feeling hungry for a couple of days a week is not going to harm you. Learn to 'own' your hunger and take control of how you deal with it.

- **If you feel you can't do it by yourself then get some support.** Encourage a friend or partner to join you on the 5:2 Diet. Having someone to talk things through with can be a real help.

- **Get moving!** Being active isn't a necessity for the 5:2 Diet to have results but as with all diets, increased activity will complement your weight loss efforts. Think about what you are doing each day: choose the stairs instead of the lift, walk to the shops instead of driving. Making small changes will not only help you burn calories but will make you feel healthier and more in control of your weight loss.

- **Don't beat yourself up!** If you have a bad day forget about it, don't feel guilty. Recognise where you went wrong and move on. Tomorrow is a new day and you can start all over again. Fast for just two days a week and you'll see results. Guaranteed!

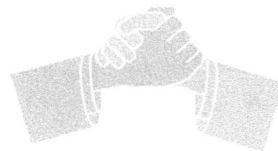

NUTRITION

All of the recipes in this collection are balanced low calorie single serving meals and snacks which should keep you feeling full on your fasting days. In any diet, it is important to balance your food between proteins, good carbs, dairy, fruit and vegetables.

- **Protein.** Keeps you feeling full and is also essential for building body tissue. Good protein sources come from meat, fish and eggs.

- **Carbohydrates.** Not all carbs are good and generally they are high in calories, which makes them difficult to include in a calorie limiting diet. Carbs are a good source of energy for your body as they are converted more easily into glucose (sugar) providing energy. Try to eat 'good carbs' which are high in fibre and nutrients e.g. whole fruits and veg, nuts, seeds, whole grain cereals, beans and legumes.

- **Dairy.** Dairy products provide you with vitamins and minerals. Cheeses can be very high in calories but other products such as low fat Greek yoghurt, crème fraiche and skimmed milk are all good.

- **Fruit & Vegetables.** Eat your five a day. There is never a better time to fill your 5 a day quota. Not only are fruit and veg very healthy, they also fill up your plate and are ideal snacks when you are feeling hungry.

CALORIE CONSCIOUS SIDE SUGGESTIONS

If you want to add an ingredient to one of our recipes here's a list of some key side vegetables, salad, noodles etc that you may find useful when working out your calories.

All calories are per 100g/3½ oz. Rice and noodle measurements are cooked weights.

	Calories		Calories
Asparagus	20	Mixed salad leaves	17
Beansprouts	20	Mushrooms	22
Brussel Sprouts	42	Pak choi/bok choy	13
Butternut Squash	45	Parsnips	70
Cabbage	30	Peas	80
Carrots	41	Peppers	40
Cauliflower:	25	Potatoes	88
Celery	14	Rocket	15
Courgette/zucchini	16	Long grain rice	140
Cucumber	15	Spinach	23
Egg noodles	62	Sweet Potato	86
Green beans	31	Sweet corn	60
Leeks	61	Tomatoes	18

STORE CUPBOARD ESSENTIALS

Our MANFOOD recipes frequently use many of the following ingredients, most of which will store for weeks in your kitchen cupboard. Stock up and you won't get caught out. Don't be afraid to substitute ingredients too and add your own twist to our meals.

Low cal cooking oil spray	Dried pasta
Tomato puree	Microwave Rice
Tomato passata	Couscous
Tinned pulses (chickpeas/blackeye beans/flageolet)	Fresh herbs - corriander, flat leaf parsley, basil, chives, oregano, mint
Lemon juice	Gnocchi
Lime juice	Straight-to-wok noodles
Thai fish sauce	Chicken & vegetable stock cubes
Pitted olives	Clear honey
Paprika	Fresh/lazy Garlic
Turmeric	Fresh/lazy ginger
Curry powder	Soy sauce
English & Dijon mustard	Worcestershire sauce
Ground Corriander	Tinned tuna (in water not brine or oil)
Crushed chilli flakes	Free-range eggs
Dried Italian herbs	Crushed sea salt
Olive Oil	Ground black pepper
Balsamic Vinegar	

ABOUT COOKNATION

CookNation is the leading publisher of innovative and practical recipe books for the modern, health-conscious cook.

CookNation titles bring together delicious, easy and practical recipes with their unique approach - making cooking for diets and healthy eating fast, simple and fun.

With a range of #1 best-selling titles - from the innovative 'Skinny' calorie-counted series, to the 5:2 Diet Recipes Collection - CookNation recipe books prove that 'Diet' can still mean 'Delicious'!

Turn to the end of this book here to browse all CookNation's recipe books. **CookNation**

MANFOOD

UNDER 200 CALORIES

BLUEBERRY BREAKFAST SMOOTHIE

180 calories per serving

Ingredients

RICH IN VITAMINS C & E

- 120ml/½ cup fat free Greek yogurt
- 1 small banana
- 50g/2oz blueberries
- Handful of ice cubes

Method

1 Peel the banana and break into 3 pieces.

2 Throw everything in the blender and blend until smooth.

3 Add more ice if you want to alter the texture.

4 That's it, breakfast done and dusted in about 30 seconds flat!

CHEFS NOTE
Use frozen blueberries if you like.

ANCHOVY & CHILLI NO-CARB SPAGHETTI

180 calories per serving

Ingredients

- 1 large courgette
- 2 tsp olive oil
- 5 anchovy fillets, drained
- ½ onion, sliced
- ½ tsp crushed chilli flakes
- 2 tsp lemon juice
- ½ tsp dried thyme
- Salt & pepper to taste

Method

1 Here's how to make your carb free spaghetti using one large courgette Either buy yourself a vegetable spiralizer or grab a potato peeler and finely 'julienne' the courgette into tiny thin slices (See page 90 if you need a bit more direction).

2 Once you've made your spaghetti get a frying pan gently heating up on the hob with the olive oil.

3 Add the anchovy fillets and onions and sauté for a few minutes until softened. Add the chilli flakes, lemon juice & thyme and continue cooking & stirring until the anchovy fillets begin to dissolve.

4 Throw in the 'spaghetti' and move around the pan for 4-6 minutes or until everything is piping hot.

5 Tip into a bowl and dig in.

CHEFS NOTE

Lets be honest....courgettes don't taste like pasta! But you'll be surprised how enjoyable vegetable spaghetti can be on your fast days.

PRAWN & BEANSPROUT GRAB LUNCH

190 calories per serving

Ingredients

- 1 carrot
- ½ cucumber, cut into batons
- 1 tbsp soy sauce
- 1 tsp brown sugar
- 1 tbsp lime juice
- ½ tsp crushed chilli flakes

- 150g/5oz cooked king prawns/jumbo shrimp
- 75g/3oz fresh beansprouts
- 1 tbsp freshly chopped coriander/cilantro
- Salt & pepper to taste

Method

1 Grab the carrot. Give it a quick peel, top & tail it and use a grater to grate the whole thing.

2 Make a simple dressing by mixing up the soy sauce, brown sugar, lime juice & chilli flakes.

3 Load the cucumber, carrot, prawns and beansprouts into a bowl, pour over the dressing and toss it really well to cover as much of the salad as possible. Throw the chopped coriander over the top and you're all set!

CHEFS NOTE
This makes a good lunchbox to take out with you, but hold off pouring over the dressing until you are ready to eat!

OATIE BREAKFAST PANCAKE

160 calories per serving

Ingredients

- 2 tbsp fine porridge oats
- 1 medium free-range egg
- 1 tsp clear honey
- ½ tsp vanilla extract
- 1 tsp low fat 'butter' spread

FIBRE RICH!

Method

1 Throw everything, except the 'butter', into a blender.

2 Give it a whizz for a few seconds until it's a smooth batter.

3 Heat up a non-stick 20cm/8 inch frying pan and add the 'butter'. Once it's melted pour in the pancake batter.

4 Gently cook for about a minute. Flip it and cook for 30-60 seconds longer or until it's cooked through.

CHEFS NOTE

This is a tasty & easy start to set you up on your fast day.

STEAMED HADDOCK & CHIVES

185 calories per serving

Ingredients

- 1 skinless haddock fillet weighing 150g/5oz
- 100g/3½oz spinach leaves
- 1 tbsp fat free crème fraiche
- 1 tsp Dijon mustard
- 1 tbsp chopped chives
- Salt & pepper to taste

Method

1 Season the fish and place in the bottom tier of a steamer. Cover with the lid and leave to steam for 5 minutes.

2 Add the spinach to the second tier of the steamer, replace the lid and steam for another 5 minutes or until the fish is cooked through.

3 Meanwhile gently heat the crème fraiche and mustard in a pan until they combine to make a sauce.

4 Arrange the spinach on a plate. Sit the fish on top, pour over the sauce and sprinkle with chives. Done.

CHEFS NOTE

If you haven't got a steamer you could poach the fish in a saucepan for 10 minutes in a little skimmed milk.

SOFT BOILED EGG & ASPARAGUS

125 calories per serving

Ingredients

- 1 large free-range egg
- 150g/5oz asparagus tips
- Salt & pepper to taste

← PERFECT START TO THE DAY

Method

1 Place the egg in a small pan and cover with cold water. Add a lid and bring to the boil on the highest heat.

2 As soon as it starts boiling (that's proper bubbles) give it 3 minutes of cooking before tipping the water out the pan. Refill with cold water and leave for a few seconds to cool the egg so that you can pick up with your hands.

3 While the egg is cooking steam the asparagus for 2-3 minutes...just give it long enough to gently cook but keep a bit of its crunch.

4 Peel the egg, lay the asparagus on a small plate and sit the egg top. Cut it in halve so that the runny yolk oozes out.

5 Add a load of salt & black pepper and eat up.

CHEFS NOTE

If you haven't got a steamer just boil the asparagus for 1-2 minutes instead.

CHEESE & SPINACH OMELETTE

195 calories per serving

Ingredients

- 2 medium free-range eggs
- 25g/1oz low fat grated cheddar cheese
- 25g/1oz spinach leaves
- Low cal cooking oil spray
- Salt & pepper to taste

LOTS OF IRON!

Method

1 Beat the eggs together in a bowl for a few seconds and season well. Add the spinach & cheese and combine.

2 Heat up the frying pan and add a little low cal spray. Pour in the eggs and cook for 2 minutes. Fold the omelette in half and cook for a minute longer or until the eggs are set.

3 Slide onto a plate or eat straight out of the pan.

CHEFS NOTE
Use a good 20cm/8inch non-stick frying pan for omelettes.

BANANA BLENDER PANCAKE

180 calories per serving

Ingredients

- 1 medium free-range egg
- 1 small banana, peeled
- ½ tsp baking powder
- ½ tsp vanilla extract
- Pinch of ground cinnamon (optional)
- 1 tsp low fat 'butter' spread

Method

1 Throw everything, except the 'butter', into a blender.

2 Give it a whizz for a few seconds until it's a smooth batter.

3 Heat up the frying pan and add the 'butter'. Once it's melted pour in the pancake batter.

4 Gently cook for about 2 minutes then turn it over and cook for about 2 minutes more.

5 Slide it out onto a plate and dig in.

CHEFS NOTE

This pancake is best cooked in a 20cm/8inch non-stick frying pan.

WATERMELON & MINT SMOOTHIE

160 calories per serving

Ingredients

- 120ml/½ cup fat free Greek yogurt
- 250g/9oz watermelon flesh, deseeded
- 3 mint leaves (use more or less to suit your taste)
- 1 tsp clear honey
- Handful ice cubes

Method

1 Throw everything in your blender and blend until smooth.

2 Add more ice if you want to alter the texture.

CHEFS NOTE

This is not a particularly thick smoothie but the sheer volume of liquid should help keep you feeling full for a while.

FRESH TOMATO EGG WHITE OMELETTE

95 calories per serving

Ingredients

- 2 egg whites from large free-range eggs
- 1 tsp low cal 'butter' spread
- 125g/4oz cherry tomatoes, chopped
- 50g/2oz rocket
- Salt & pepper to taste

Method

1 Beat the eggs whites together in a bowl for a few seconds and season well.

2 Heat up the frying pan and melt the 'butter'. Pour in the eggs and cook for a minute. Flip and cook for a minute longer or until the eggs are set.

3 Slide onto a plate, load the fresh tomatoes and rocket into the middle and fold.

CHEFS NOTE

Use a good quality 20cm/8inch non-stick frying pan for cooking one-person omelettes.

EGG FRIED SPINACH 'RICE'

178 calories per serving

Ingredients

- 200g/7oz cauliflower florets
- 1 tsp olive oil
- ½ onion, chopped
- 1 garlic clove, crushed
- 1 tsp soy sauce
- 1 small free-range egg
- 50g/2oz spinach

Method

1 Place the cauliflower florets in a food processor and pulse a few times until the cauliflower is the size of rice grains.

2 Place the 'rice' in a microwavable dish, cover and cook on full power for about 2 minutes or until the 'rice' is piping hot. When it's done put to one side

3 Whilst the rice is cooking heat the oil in a frying pan and sauté the onion and garlic for a few minutes until the onions soften. Add the 'rice to the pan along with the soy sauce and move around well.

4 Break the egg into the centre and quickly stir-fry

until you see the egg 'set'. Add the spinach and cook for a further 30 seconds.

5 Tip into a bowl and eat your fakeaway fried rice straight away!

CHEFS NOTE

The spinach will not be fully wilted. Cook for longer if that's how you like it.

MANFOOD

SOUPS UNDER 250 CALORIES

CARROT & CRUSHED CHILLI SOUP

170 calories per serving

Ingredients

- 1 tsp olive oil
- ½ onion, sliced
- ½ garlic clove, crushed
- 100g/3½oz carrots, peeled & chopped
- 75g/3oz potatoes, peeled & chopped
- 370ml/1½ cups low sodium vegetable stock
- ½ tsp crushed chilli flakes
- Salt & pepper to taste

Method

1 Get the olive oil warming up in a non-stick saucepan on a gentle heat.

2 Throw in the onions, garlic, carrots and potatoes and gently sauté for 4-5 minutes or until everything begins to soften up.

3 Add the hot stock, bring to the boil, cover and leave to simmer for 10 minutes or until the vegetables are tender.

4 Tip the hot soup into a blender and blend until smooth, take care with the hot liquid and cover properly with the lid. Pour into a bowl and sprinkle with the crushed chillies.

CHEFS NOTE
Add a swirl of milk if you've got a few calories to spare.

EASY VEGGIE SOUP

210 calories per serving

Ingredients

- 1 tsp olive oil
- ½ onion, sliced
- 75g/3oz carrots, peeled & chopped
- 75g/3oz parsnips, peeled & chopped
- 75g/3oz turnips, peeled & chopped
- 75g/3oz potatoes, peeled & chopped
- 370/1½ cups low sodium vegetable stock
- Salt & pepper to taste

Method

1 Get the olive oil warming up in a non-stick saucepan on a gentle heat.

2 Throw in all the vegetables and gently sauté for 4-5 minutes or until everything begins to soften up.

3 Add the hot stock, bring to the boil, cover and leave to simmer for 10 minutes or until the vegetables are tender.

4 Tip the hot soup into a blender and blend until smooth.

CHEFS NOTE

Use any root vegetables you have to hand. Many shops sell ready prepared soup mixes.

CHILLED MELON SOUP

120 calories per serving

Ingredients

- Flesh of ½ cantaloupe melon
- 60ml/¼ cup fresh orange juice
- 2 large fresh mint leaves

FRESH & LIGHT!

Method

1 This chilled soup couldn't be any easier...just load the lot into a blender and blend until smooth.

2 Either eat it straight away or place it in the fridge for later.

CHEFS NOTE

Don't try and peel the melon. Just cut it in half. Discard the seeds and scoop out the flesh with a large spoon.

SPICY AVOCADO & CUCUMBER SOUP

170 calories per serving

Ingredients

HEALTHY FATS!

- ½ cucumber
- 1 stalk of celery
- ½ avocado
- ½ tsp cayenne pepper
- Pinch of sea salt

Method

1 Busting with good fats this is another light and simple chilled soup.

2 Chop up the cucumber and celery. Stone the avocado and scoop out the flesh.

3 Place everything into a blender and blend until smooth (add a little water if you need to get the consistency right).

4 Either eat it straight away or place it in the fridge for later.

CHEFS NOTE

This is also handy as a savoury smoothie, which you can tip into a drinks container and take to work.

SWEET POTATO & COCONUT CREAM SOUP

240 calories per serving

Ingredients

- 1 tsp olive oil
- ½ onion, sliced
- ½ garlic clove, crushed
- 150g/5oz sweet potatoes, peeled & chopped
- 1 tbsp coconut cream
- 250ml/1 cup low sodium vegetable stock
- 2 tsp freshly chopped parsley
- Salt & pepper to taste

Method

1 Get the olive oil warming up in a non-stick saucepan on a gentle heat.

2 Throw in the onions, garlic & sweet potatoes and gently sauté for 4-5 minutes or until everything begins to soften up.

3 Add the hot stock, bring to the boil, cover and leave to simmer for 10 minutes or until the vegetables are tender.

4 Stir through the coconut cream, tip the hot soup into a blender and blend until smooth.

5 Pour into a bowl, sprinkle with parsley and dive in.

CHEFS NOTE
Use flat leaf parsley rather than the curly variety.

CHICKEN & SWEETCORN SOUP

220 calories per serving

Ingredients

- ½ onion, sliced
- ½ garlic clove, crushed
- 100g/3½oz sweetcorn
- 250ml/1 cup low sodium vegetable stock
- 75g/3oz cooked chicken breast, shredded
- Salt & pepper to taste

Method

1 Place the onion, garlic, sweetcorn & hot stock in a pan.

2 Bring to the boil, cover and leave to simmer for about 5 minutes.

3 Tip into a blender or food processor and pulse a couple of times so you get a chunky textured soup.

4 Get the soup back into the pan and add the shredded chicken. Warm through for a few minutes until everything is piping hot. Add some salt & pepper and serve.

CHEFS NOTE
Add more stock if you want a thinner base to the soup.

LEAN, GREEN SOUP

98 calories per serving

Ingredients

- 1 tsp olive oil
- 1 onion, sliced
- ½ garlic clove, crushed
- 75g/3oz spinach
- 250ml/1 cup low sodium vegetable stock
- 1 tbsp low fat single cream
- 25g/1oz watercress
- Salt & pepper to taste

Method

1 Get the olive oil warming up in a non-stick saucepan on a gentle heat.

2 Throw in the onions & garlic and gently sauté for 4-5 minutes or until the onions soften up.

3 Add the spinach & hot stock. Bring to the boil, cover and leave to simmer for 5 minutes.

4 Tip the hot soup into a blender and blend until smooth. Pour into a bowl and gently swirl the cream through. Sit the watercress on top and dig in.

CHEFS NOTE

Adding the watercress when serving gives the soup a nice fresh 'crunch'.

IRISH POTATO SOUP

195 calories per serving

Ingredients

- 1 tsp olive oil
- ½ onion, sliced
- 200g/7oz potatoes, peeled & diced
- 1 tsp dried rosemary
- 250ml/1 cup low sodium vegetable stock
- Salt & pepper to taste

Method

1 Get the olive oil warming up in a non-stick saucepan on a gentle heat.

2 Throw in the onions, potatoes & rosemary and gently sauté for 4-5 minutes or until everything starts to soften up.

3 Add the hot stock, bring to the boil, cover and leave to simmer for 10 minutes.

4 Tip the hot soup into a blender and blend until smooth (add more stock or hot water if it's too thick). Pour into a bowl and season with plenty of black pepper.

CHEFS NOTE

Add a dash of milk if you want it a little creamier.

SPICY CRAB NOODLE SOUP

160 calories per serving

Ingredients

- ½ onion, sliced
- ½ tsp crushed chilli flakes
- 25g/1oz dried egg noodles
- 250ml/1 cup low sodium vegetable stock
- 50g/2oz tinned crab meat
- Salt & pepper to taste

Method

1 Add the onions, chilli flakes, noodles and hot stock to a saucepan. Bring to the boil, cover and leave to simmer for 4-5 minutes or until the noodles are cooked.

2 Flake the crabmeat with a fork and add to the soup, warm through for a few minutes until everything is piping hot.

3 Slice the spring onions thinly lengthways to make ribbons.

4 Tip the soup into a bowl and scatter the spring onions on top. Job done.

CHEFS NOTE
Break the noodles up a bit before cooking, it'll make the soup easier to eat with a spoon.

CAULIFLOWER SOUP

220 calories per serving

Ingredients

- 1 tsp olive oil
- ½ onion, sliced
- 300g/11oz cauliflower florets, chopped
- 75g/3oz potatoes, peeled & diced
- 250ml/1 cup low sodium vegetable stock
- 15g/½oz low fat grated cheddar cheese
- Salt & pepper to taste

Method

1 Get the olive oil warming up in a non-stick saucepan on a gentle heat.

2 Throw in the onions, cauliflower and potatoes and gently sauté for 4-5 minutes or until everything starts to soften up.

3 Add the hot stock, bring to the boil, cover and leave to simmer for 10 minutes.

4 Tip the soup into a blender and blend until smooth (add more stock or water if it's too thick). Pour into a bowl, sprinkle the cheese on top and season with plenty of black pepper.

CHEFS NOTE

Use low fat mature cheddar if you can.

MANFOOD

UNDER 300 CALORIES

PRAWN & ROCKET SALAD

250 calories per serving

Ingredients

- 125g/4oz cooked king prawns
- ½ red pepper, deseeded & sliced
- ½ red onion, sliced
- ½ tsp crushed chilli flakes
- ½ tsp ground cumin
- 75g/3oz tinned sweetcorn, drained

- 4 cherry tomatoes, chopped
- 1 tbsp lime juice
- 1 baby gem lettuce, shredded
- 50g/2oz rocket
- Salt & pepper to taste

Method

1 Mix the prawns, peppers, onion, crushed chilli, cumin, sweetcorn, tomatoes and lime juice in a bowl and combine really well with plenty of salt and pepper.

2 Add the shredded lettuce & rocket, toss it around and tip onto your plate.

3 That's it. Easy, fresh and ready in minutes.

CHEFS NOTE

If you aren't mad on prawns try shredded chicken instead.

GRILLED CHICKEN & ASPARAGUS

290 calories per serving

Ingredients

- 1 skinless chicken breast weighing 125g/4oz
- 200g/7oz asparagus tips
- 1 tbsp fat free Greek yogurt
- 1 tsp Dijon mustard
- 1 tsp clear honey
- 50g/2oz rocket
- Low cal cooking oil spray
- Salt & pepper to taste

Method

1 Preheat the grill to a medium/high heat.

2 Bash the chicken a few times with a rolling pin so it's tender. Season, spray with a little low cal oil and cook under the hot grill for 5 minutes.

3 Place the asparagus beside the chicken and spray with a bit of oil. Get everything back under the grill and cook for another 5-7 minutes or until the chicken is cooked through and the asparagus is tender.

4 When the chicken is ready cut it into thick slices. Put to one side and mix together the yogurt, mustard and honey.

5 Load the chicken slices onto the rocket with the asparagus on the side. Pour the yogurt dressing over the chicken and get stuck in.

CHEFS NOTE

Chicken is a great low fat source of protein.

TURKEY & TOMATO KEBABS

240 calories per serving

Ingredients

- 150g/5oz turkey breast, cubed
- 150g/5oz whole cherry tomatoes
- 150g/5oz whole button mushrooms
- 1 tbsp soy sauce
- 1 tsp clear honey
- 1 garlic clove, crushed
- Metal kebab sticks
- Low cal cooking oil spray
- Salt & pepper to taste

Method

1 Preheat the grill to a medium/high heat.

2 Place the cubed turkey, tomatoes, mushrooms, soy sauce, honey & garlic in a bowl and give them a good mix.

3 Place the turkey, tomatoes and mushrooms onto wooden skewers in turn to make a couple of kebabs.

4 Give them a little spray of low cal oil and stick under the grill. Cook for about 10 minutes (turning now and again) or until the turkey is cooked through.

CHEFS NOTE
Serve with a salad if you want to bulk this up a bit.

SWEET CHILLI SALMON

Ingredients

- 1 skinless salmon fillet weighing 150g/5oz
- 2 tsp sweet chilli sauce
- 1 tbsp soy sauce

- 75g/3oz mixed salad leaves
- Salt & pepper to taste

Method

1 Preheat the oven to 200C/400F/Gas 6.

2 Mix the sweet chilli sauce and soy sauce together. Place the salmon fillet in an ovenproof dish and brush the sauce all over it.

3 Put the salmon in the preheated oven and cook for about 20 minutes or until fully cooked through.

4 When it's ready place it on top of the salad leaves and serve.

CHEFS NOTE
You can tell the salmon is ready when the flesh gently flakes with a fork.

PINEAPPLE CHICKEN

295 calories per serving

Ingredients

- 1 skinless chicken breast weighing 125g/4oz
- 1 small bunch fresh coriander/cilantro
- 4 spring onions/scallions
- 1 tsp lime juice

- 100g/3½oz tinned pineapple chunks
- ½ tsp crushed chilli flakes
- 125g/4oz green beans
- Low cal cooking oil spray
- Salt & pepper to taste

Method

1 Preheat the grill to a medium/high heat.

2 Bash the chicken a few times with a rolling pin to make it tender. Season, spray with a little low cal oil and cook under the hot grill for about 10-12 minutes or until it's cooked through.

3 While the chicken is cooking add the fresh coriander, spring onions, lime juice, pineapple & chilli flakes to a food processor and pulse for a few seconds to make a chunky fruit salsa.

4 Meanwhile plunge the beans into a pan of salted boiling water and cook for just 2 minutes – you want them to still be crunchy.

5 When the chicken is ready sit it on a plate with the green beans on the side and tip the salsa over the top of the meat. Sit down and eat up.

CHEFS NOTE

Use salad or any other greens you like to accompany the chicken if you don't have green beans to hand.

FRESH FRUIT BREAKFAST

260 calories per serving

Ingredients

← **ANTIOXIDANT RICH!**

- 200g/7oz fresh strawberries
- 1 whole pomegranate
- 1 whole kiwi
- 2 tbsp fat free Greek yogurt
- 1 tsp clear honey

Method

1 Get rid of the green tops and slice the strawberries in half.

2 Release the seeds from the pomegranate by cutting it in half, and banging each halve hard with the back of a spoon until the seeds come flying out.

3 Peel the kiwi and cube it up.

4 Load all the fruit into a bowl. Dollop with yogurt and drizzle the honey over the top. Simple and delicious!

CHEFS NOTE
Busting with fresh goodness this breakfast will set you up for the day.

SIMPLE HERBED TABBOULEH

210 calories per serving

Ingredients

- 50g/2oz bulgur wheat
- 250ml/1 cup hot vegetable stock
- 3 spring onions/scallions
- 6 cherry tomatoes
- 2 tsp lemon juice
- 1 tbsp freshly chopped basil
- 1 tbsp freshly chopped mint
- Salt & pepper to taste

Method

1 Put the bulgur wheat and stock in a saucepan, cover and cook for about 20-25 minutes or until it's tender. (Add more stock or water if you need to and when it's ready drain off any excess liquid).

2 While the wheat is cooking get on with chopping up the spring onions and cherry tomatoes and put to one side.

3 Once the bulgur wheat is ready fluff it up with a fork. Add the chopped onions and tomatoes, lemon juice and the fresh herbs. Work it around really well, season and serve.

CHEFS NOTE

Add extra lemon juice and more fresh herbs if you want.

BAKED LEMON CHICKEN

299 calories per serving

Ingredients

- 1 skinless chicken breast weighing 150g/5oz
- ½ lemon, thinly sliced
- 1 courgette, thinly sliced lengthways
- ½ onion, sliced

- 75g/3oz watercress
- Low cal cooking oil spray
- Salt & pepper to taste

Method

1 Preheat the oven to 200C/400F/Gas 6.

2 Place the chicken breast on a large piece of tin foil and cover with lemon slices.

3 Lay the courgettes slices and chopped onions on top of the chicken and fold the foil into a loose parcel leaving enough room for the steam to circulate freely around the top and sides of the chicken and courgettes.

4 Place in oven and cook for about 25-30 minutes or until the chicken fully cooked through.

5 When it's ready place everything on top of the watercress, fish out the lemon slices and serve.

CHEFS NOTE
You could bake some whole garlic cloves with this. Crush them and serve over the top of the chicken.

HOISIN STEAK

280 calories per serving

Ingredients

- 50g/2oz mushrooms, sliced
- 50g/2oz green beans, halved
- 1 garlic clove, crushed
- ½ onion, sliced
- 1 tbsp hoisin sauce

- 1 tbsp soy sauce
- 100g/3½oz trimmed sirloin steak
- Low cal cooking oil spray
- Salt & pepper to taste

Method

1 Throw the mushrooms, beans, garlic & onion in a frying pan with some low cal spray and gently sauté for 3 minutes (add a splash of water to the pan if you need to loosen it up).

2 Slice the steak up into thick strips and add to the pan along with the hoisin & soy sauce. Stir-fry for two minutes (or less if you prefer your steak rare).

3 Tip the lot into a bowl and grab a fork.

CHEFS NOTE
Got some spring onions? Roughly chop them and sprinkle over the top.

GRILLED COD & CHERRY TOMATOES

230 calories per serving

Ingredients

- 1 skinless cod fillet weighing 150g/5oz
- ½ garlic clove, crushed
- 1 tsp freshly chopped rosemary
- ½ tsp brown sugar
- 6 cherry tomatoes, halved

- 75g/3oz spinach
- 1 tsp low fat mayonnaise
- Low cal cooking oil spray
- Salt & pepper to taste

Method

1 Preheat the grill to a medium/high heat and season the cod fillet.

2 Mix the garlic, rosemary, sugar and tomatoes together in a bowl.

3 Spray the cod with a little low cal cooking oil and place under the preheated grill along with the tomatoes.

4 Grill for about 8 minutes or until the fish is cooked through.

5 Sit the raw spinach leaves on a plate. Tip the fish and tomatoes over and eat up.

CHEFS NOTE

Cod is good but any firm white fish fillet will work well.

FIVE SPICE SCALLOPS

210 calories per serving

Ingredients

- 1 garlic clove, crushed
- 1 tbsp soy sauce
- 1 tsp Chinese five spice powder
- ½ tsp crushed chillies
- 50g/2oz asparagus tips, halved
- 4 spring onions/scallions, chopped
- 75g/3oz spinach leaves
- 6 shelled, prepared fresh scallops
- Lime wedges to serve
- Low cal cooking oil spray
- Salt & pepper to taste

Method

1 First make a dressing by mixing together the garlic, soy sauce, five spice powder & crushed chillies.

2 Get a frying pan gently heating up with a little low cal spray. Place the scallops in there and cook for a minute. Add the asparagus, spring onions & dressing and cook on a medium heat for about 2-3 minutes or until the scallops are cooked through (add a splash of water to the pan if you need to loosen it up).

3 At the last minute load the spinach into the pan and give it a quick stir to combine. Tip the lot out into a bowl and eat up!

CHEFS NOTE
If you like your spinach wilted add to the pan when you add the asparagus and spring onions.

SAVOURY STEAMED LENTILS & GREEN BEANS

250 calories per serving

Ingredients

- 50g/2oz red split lentils
- 120ml/½ cup vegetable stock
- 75g/3oz green beans, roughly chopped
- ½ carrot, grated
- 6 spring onions, finely sliced
- 1 tbsp soy sauce
- 1 tbsp lemon juice
- Salt & pepper to taste

Method

1 Throw the lentils & stock into a steam-proof glass bowl.

2 Place the bowl in the bottom tier of a steamer. Cover the steamer with the lid and steam for 45 minutes. (Stir once or twice during cooking and add additional stock if you need to).

3 Place the green beans on top of the lentils, replace the lid and steam for another 10 minutes or until the lentils and beans are tender and cooked through.

4 Tip the lentils into a bowl, pile the grated carrot and spring onions on top. Mix together the soy sauce & lemon juice and get that over the lentils too. Job done.

CHEFS NOTE
Cooking this in the steamer means you can forget about it and get on with something else but make sure there's plenty of water in the steamer.

CHILLI & BROCCOLI LINGUINE

270 calories per serving

Ingredients

- 50g/2oz linguine
- 1 garlic clove, crushed
- 150g/5oz tenderstem broccoli, chopped
- ½ onion, chopped
- 1 tsp anchovy paste
- 2 tsp water
- ½ tsp crushed chilli flakes
- Low cal cooking oil spray
- Salt & pepper to taste

Method

1 Put the pasta in a pan of salted boiling water. Cover and cook for about 10 minutes or until it's tender.

2 Meanwhile gently sauté the garlic, chopped broccoli and onions in a little low cal spray for a few minutes until softened (add a splash of water to the pan if you need to loosen it up).

3 Mix together the anchovy paste and water and add this to the pan along with the chilli flakes. When the pasta is ready toss the anchovy broccoli through it and serve up.

CHEFS NOTE
Anchovy paste is handy but tinned anchovy fillets will work just as well.

TURKEY & PEANUT BUTTER NOODLES

295 calories per serving

Ingredients

- 50g/2oz dried fine egg noodles
- ½ vegetable stock cube
- ½ tsp crushed chilli flakes
- 2 tsp low fat peanut butter
- 1 tbsp soy sauce
- 1 tbsp lime juice

- 1 tbsp boiling water
- 4 spring onions/scallions, chopped
- 1 red pepper, deseeded & sliced
- 75g/3oz cooked turkey breast, thinly sliced
- Salt & pepper to taste

Method

1 Crumble the stock in a pan of boiling water and stir to dissolve. Add the egg noodles, cover and leave to cook on the hob for a few minutes while you get busy with the other bits.

2 Mix up the chilli flakes, peanut butter, soy sauce, lime juice and boiling water. (The heat of the water should loosen the peanut butter up).

3 Drain the noodles and throw these in a bowl with the spring onions, peppers and sliced turkey. Toss through the peanut better dressing and grab yourself a fork.

CHEFS NOTE
Add more chilli flakes if you want to ramp up the 'heat'.

GNOCCHI & GARLIC

230 calories per serving

Ingredients

- 100g/3½oz gnocchi
- 2 tsp low fat 'butter' spread
- 1 garlic clove crushed

- 50g/2oz watercress
- 1 tsp grated Parmesan cheese
- Salt & pepper to taste

Method

1 Add the gnocchi to a pan of salted boiling water. Lower the heat and leave to cook for 2-3 minutes or until the gnocchi rises to the top of the pan.

2 Meanwhile melt the 'butter' in a frying pan along with the crushed garlic.

3 Drain the gnocchi and tip it into the melted garlic butter. Move around the pan really well for a minute or two to cover each dumpling in the garlic butter.

4 Tip into a bowl. Sprinkle over the Parmesan, sit the watercress on top and eat up.

CHEFS NOTE
Toss the watercress through the gnocchi if you prefer to eat it that way.

HAM & EGGS

240 calories per serving

Ingredients

- 75g/3oz asparagus tips
- 1 large free-range egg
- 2 slices Parma ham

- 1 slice wholemeal bread
- Low cal cooking oil spray
- Salt & pepper to taste

Method

1 Preheat the grill to medium and boil a kettle of water.

2 Place the asparagus on the rack and spray with a bit of oil. Get it under the grill and cook for about 5 minutes or until the asparagus is tender.

3 Meanwhile warm a pan on the hob and pour in a couple of inches of boiling water. Crack the egg into the pan and leave to poach while the asparagus grills. Put the bread into the toaster for a couple of minutes too.

4 When the egg is cooked to your liking, remove it from the pan and put it on a bit of kitchen roll to drain off the excess water.

5 The next job is to get everything piled up together. Start with the toast, tip over the asparagus and sit the Parma ham on top. Finish with a poached egg and plenty of freshly ground black pepper.

CHEFS NOTE

Any type of prosciutto ham will do the job, add a dash of hot sauce to the egg if you like.

TURKEY CURRY & 'RICE'

290 calories per serving

Ingredients

- ½ onion, chopped
- 75g/3oz peas
- 1 garlic clove, crushed
- 125g/4oz turkey breast, sliced
- 1 tbsp hot curry powder
- **1 portion cauliflower rice** (see page 90 for recipe)

- 1 tbsp chopped sultanas
- 2 tbsp low far Greek yogurt
- 1 tbsp freshly chopped coriander/cilantro
- Low cal cooking oil spray
- Salt & pepper to taste

Method

1 Get the onions, peas and garlic gently cooking in a frying pan with some low cal spray. Gently sauté for a couple of minutes and then add the turkey and curry powder along with a tablespoon of water to keep the pan loose.

2 Stir well and cook for a few minutes until the turkey is cooked thorough.

3 Meanwhile get your cauliflower rice nice & hot and combine with chopped sultanas.

4 Remove the turkey pan from the heat and stir through the yoghurt.

5 Tip the 'rice' into a shallow bowl. Get the curry over the top and sprinkle with freshly chopped coriander.

CHEFS NOTE
Keep portions of cauliflower rice handy as these make a great 'skinny' alternative to real rice.

PESTO CHICKEN WITH FAKE SPAGHETTI

299 calories per serving

Ingredients

- 1 large courgette
- 1 tbsp green pesto sauce
- 100g/3½oz cooked chicken breast, shredded

- 2 tsp grated Parmesan cheese
- Low cal cooking oil spray
- Salt & pepper to taste

Method

1 This is where things get a bit clever on the carb front.... Your first job is to transform the courgette into 'spaghetti'. You can do this a couple of ways: the first option is to buy yourself a vegetable spiralizer which will make your life easy or grab a potato peeler and finely 'julienne' the courgette into tiny thin slices (see page 90 if you need a bit more direction).

2 When you've made your spaghetti get a frying pan gently heating up on the hob. Throw in the spaghetti with a little low cal spray and move about the pan for a couple of minutes (add a splash of water to the pan if you need to loosen it up).

3 Combine the shredded chicken with the pesto sauce and add this to the pan too. Mix really well and continue cooking until everything is piping hot.

4 Tip into a bowl, sprinkle over the cheese and dig in.

CHEFS NOTE

Treat yourself to a vegetable spiralizer gadget and you'll find lots of new ways to cut down your carbs.

MINTED CHICKEN COUSCOUS

298 calories per serving

Ingredients

- 50g/2oz couscous
- 80ml/⅓ cup boiling hot chicken stock
- 1 tbsp lemon juice
- 1 tsp olive oil
- 1 tbsp water
- 1 tsp white wine or cider vinegar
- ½ cucumber, finely diced
- 2 tbsp freshly chopped mint
- 50g/2oz cooked chicken breast, shredded
- Salt & pepper to taste

Method

1 Place the couscous and stock in a bowl, cover and leave for 3 minutes.

2 Meanwhile mix together the lemon juice, olive oil, water and vinegar to make a simple vinaigrette. Add the cucumber, mint & chicken and combine really well.

3 When the couscous is ready fluff it up with a fork and load the dressed chicken over the top. Eat it straight away or let it cool and bang it in the fridge for later.

CHEFS NOTE
This is also good with the dressed chicken tossed through the couscous rather than piled on top.

SEA BASS LUNCH

260 calories per serving

Ingredients

- ½ onion, chopped
- 1 garlic clove, crushed
- 1 fresh sea bass fillet weighing 150g/5oz
- 50g/2oz sugar snap peas
- 125g/4oz cherry tomatoes, halved
- 2 tsp low fat mayonnaise
- 50g/2oz rocket
- Low cal cooking oil spray
- Salt & pepper to taste

Method

1 Place a frying pan on a medium heat with a little low cal spray.

2 Sauté the onions and garlic for a few minutes until softened (add a splash of water to the pan if you need to loosen it up).

3 Season the sea bass fillet and add to the pan along with the sugar snap peas & tomatoes.

4 Fry for about 6 minutes or until the fish is cooked through (turn the fish after 3 minutes).

5 Remove everything from the pan piece by piece and arrange on the plate with the rocket and mayo - don't just tip it out, you want it to look as good as it tastes!

CHEFS NOTE
The sea bass fillet may need less time depending on thickness, keep an eye on it.

MANFOOD

UNDER 400 CALORIES

PRAWN & PAK CHOI NOODLES

340 calories per serving

Ingredients

- ½ onion, chopped
- 1 tsp freshly grated ginger
- 1 garlic clove, crushed
- 125g/4oz raw shelled king prawns
- 2 tsp soy sauce
- 50g/2oz dried fine egg noodles
- ½ vegetable stock cube
- 1 large pak choi/bok choi , shredded
- Low cal cooking oil spray
- Salt & pepper to taste

Method

1 Gently sauté the onions, ginger, garlic, prawns & soy sauce in a non-stick saucepan with a little low cal oil for about 5-8 minutes or until the onions soften up and the prawns are cooked through (add a splash of water to the pan if you need to).

2 Meanwhile crumble the stock in a pan of boiling water and stir to dissolve. Add the egg noodles & pak choi and leave to cook on the hob for a few minutes until the noodles are tender.

3 Drain the noodles and throw everything into the pan with the prawns. Combine together and tip into a bowl. Job done.

CHEFS NOTE
Sprinkle over some thinly sliced chillies if you fancy it.

TEX MEX BEANS & EGGS

350 calories per serving

Ingredients

- ½ red onion
- 2 vine ripened plum tomatoes
- 1 garlic clove
- 3 tsp lime juice
- ½ red chilli

- 100g/3½oz tinned black beans
- ½ tsp ground cumin & paprika
- 2 medium free-range eggs
- 125g/4oz spinach
- Salt & pepper to taste

Method

1 The first job is to put together a simple salsa: make your life easy by digging out the food processor and throwing in the onion, tomatoes, garlic, 2 tsp lime juice & chilli. Pulse a few times until it's finely chopped....or do it the old fashioned way and chop everything up yourself. Season with a good pinch of salt and pepper.

2 Meanwhile drain and rinse the black beans. Throw these in a bowl with the cumin and paprika and mash them up a bit with the back of a fork and the other teaspoon of lime juice. Set to one side and get on with the eggs.

3 Heat up the frying pan and add a little low cal spray. Break the eggs into the pan, cover and fry for a few minutes or until the eggs are set.

4 Now it's time to bring it all together. Lay out the spinach. Pile the beans on top with the salsa on the side. Tip the eggs over the beans and get stuck in.

CHEFS NOTE
Use a decent non-stick frying pan to make sure your eggs don't get 'stuck'.

SPICY TUNA & RICE SALAD

380 calories per serving

Ingredients

- 50g/2oz microwave rice
- ½ red pepper, deseeded & sliced
- ½ red onion, sliced
- ½ tsp crushed chilli flakes
- 4 cherry tomatoes, halved
- ½ garlic clove, crushed

- 1 tsp olive oil
- 1 tbsp lime juice
- 75g/3oz tinned tuna, drained
- 50g/2oz tinned kidney beans, drained & rinsed
- Salt & pepper to taste

Method

1 Get the rice cooked in the microwave and leave to cool. Check the packet instructions (it usually takes about 1-2 minutes).

2 Meanwhile put all the other ingredients in a bowl and combine really well to make a salad.

3 When the rice is cool toss is through the salad. Pile onto your plate and get stuck in.

CHEFS NOTE
Use tuna that has been stored in spring water rather than oil.

NUOC MAM CHAM

370 calories per serving

Ingredients

- 125g/5oz microwave rice
- ½ onion, chopped
- 2 garlic cloves
- 1 red chilli (leave the seeds in)
- 2 tbsp lime juice
- 2 tbsp fish sauce
- 2 tsp caster sugar
- 75g/3oz cooked chicken breast, shredded
- Low cal cooking oil spray
- Salt & pepper to taste

Method

1 Get the rice cooked in the microwave and leave to cool. Check the packet instructions (it usually takes about 1-2 minutes).

2 Heat up a frying pan with a little low cal spray and start sautéing the onions for a few minutes until softened (add a splash of water to the pan if you need to loosen it up).

3 While the onions are cooking toss in the garlic cloves, chilli, lime juice, fish sauce and caster sugar in a food processor and whizz to make a spicy, sweet & sour dressing.

4 Tip the cooked rice and shredded chicken into the pan with the onions and warm for a few minutes until everything is piping hot.

5 Load the chicken & rice into a bowl and drizzle the dressing over the top. Don't hang about...dig straight in.

CHEFS NOTE

This Vietnamese dish will blow your socks off, balance the chilli, lime and sugar to suit your own taste.

PAN FRIED TUNA

370 calories per serving

Ingredients

- 50g/2oz couscous
- 1 tbsp soy sauce
- 1 tsp freshly grated ginger
- 2 spring onions/scallions, finely chopped
- 1 fresh tuna fillet weighing 150g/5oz
- 1 pak choi/bok choi, quartered
- 50g/2oz sugar snap peas
- 1 tbsp balsamic vinegar
- Low cal cooking oil spray
- Salt & pepper to taste

Method

1 First make a dressing by mixing together the soy sauce, ginger & finely chopped spring onions.

2 Place a frying pan on a medium/high heat with a little low cal spray. Season the tuna fillet and add to the pan along with the pak choi and peas. Pour the balsamic vinegar over the top of the fillet and cook the tuna for 2 minutes each side. (Keep the vegetables moving around the pan and add a splash of water if you need to).

3 Remove the tuna from the pan and leave to rest but carry on cooking the veg for a minute longer.

4 Thinly slice the tuna and arrange on a plate with the pak choi and peas on the side. Drizzle the soy sauce dressing all over the tuna slices and get stuck in!

CHEFS NOTE

Reduce the cooking time if you prefer your tuna particularly rare.

PERSIAN QUINOA

315 calories per serving

Ingredients

- 50g/2oz quinoa
- 250ml/1 cup hot vegetable stock
- 1 whole pomegranate
- 2 tsp lemon juice
- 1 carrot, grated
- 2 tbsp freshly chopped mint
- Salt & pepper to taste

Method

1 Quinoa is an alternative to rice and looks a bit like couscous. It's a complete protein packed with all the essential amino acids your body needs! Put the quinoa and stock in a saucepan, cover and cook for about 20 minutes or until it's tender. (Add more stock or water if you need to and when it's ready drain off any excess liquid).

2 While the quinoa is cooking get the seeds out of the pomegranate. To do this just cut the fruit in half, place face down on a chopping board and bang the back of each halve hard with a spoon. The seeds should come shooting out, pick out any that are left in the rind.

3 Once the quinoa is ready fluff it up with a fork and combine it with the pomegranate seeds, lemon juice and mint. Pile the grated carrot on top and it's job done.

CHEFS NOTE

Originally native to Persia pomegranates are rich in vitamins C & D.

CHICKEN NOODLE SALAD

395 calories per serving

Ingredients

- 50g/2oz dried fine egg noodles
- ½ vegetable stock cube
- ½ cucumber
- ½ red onion
- 4 spring onions/scallions
- 75g/4oz cooked chicken breast, shredded
- ½ tsp crushed chilli flakes
- 1 tsp sesame oil
- Small bunch fresh coriander/cilantro, chopped
- 1 tbsp chopped peanuts
- Salt & pepper to taste

Method

1 Crumble the stock in a pan of boiling water and stir to dissolve. Add the egg noodles, cover and leave to cook on the hob for a few minutes while you make the rest of the salad.

2 Cube up the cucumber and thinly slice the red onion and the spring onions. Throw these in a bowl with the shredded chicken and chilli flakes.

3 Drain the noodles, rinse in cold water and quickly stir through the sesame oil. Toss the noodles and fresh coriander with the chicken and onions.

4 Sprinkle with the chopped peanuts and eat straight away.

CHEFS NOTE
Use prawns instead of chicken if you like.

PARMA HAM & SPINACH SALAD

355 calories per serving

Ingredients

- 3 slices Parma ham
- 1 red pepper, deseeded & sliced
- 1 red onion, sliced
- 1 tsp grated ginger
- ½ tsp ground cumin
- 200g/7oz fresh spinach leaves
- Low cal cooking oil spray
- Salt & pepper to taste

Method

1 Throw the peppers, sliced onion, ginger & cumin in a frying pan with some low cal spray and gently sauté for about five minutes until things start to soften up (add a splash of water to the pan if you need to).

2 Get the spinach leaves set up in a shallow bowl and tip the cooked peppers and onions over.

3 Pile the shredded Parma ham on top and get stuck in.

CHEFS NOTE
If you haven't got any cumin use curry powder instead.

ROCKET, GRAPEFRUIT & PRAWNS

380 calories per serving

Ingredients

- ½ pink grapefruit
- 1 tbsp lime juice
- 1 tbsp fish sauce
- 1 tsp brown sugar
- ½ tsp crushed chilli flakes
- 1 tbsp soy sauce

- 150g/5oz cooked king prawns/jumbo shrimp
- 125g/4oz rocket
- ½ avocado, sliced
- 1 tbsp fresh mint, finely chopped
- Salt & pepper to taste

Method

1 Split the grapefruit into segments and cut each segment into three bits.

2 Mix together the lime juice, fish sauce, sugar, chilli flakes & soy sauce in a bowl. Add the prawns and combine well.

3 Pile the prawns (and any left over dressing) and grapefruit over the rocket leaves, place the avocado slices on top and sprinkle with the chopped mint.

4 Grab your fork and dig in.

CHEFS NOTE

Don't try peeling the avocado. Just split it in half with a knife, dig out the stone and get the flesh out with a big spoon.

CHERRY TOMATO & CHICKEN COUSCOUS

330 calories per serving

Ingredients

- 100g/3½oz cooked chicken breast, sliced
- 50g/2oz tinned chickpeas, drained
- 75g/3oz cherry tomatoes, halved
- 1 tbsp lemon juice
- 1 tbsp fresh basil, chopped
- 50g/2oz couscous
- 80ml/⅓ cup boiling hot chicken stock
- Low cal cooking oil spray
- Salt & pepper to taste

Method

1 Mix the chicken, chickpeas, cherry tomatoes, lemon & basil together. Put to one side while you make the other stuff.

2 Place the couscous and stock in a bowl, cover and leave for 3 minutes. When it's done fluff up with a fork.

3 Toss the lemon chicken, chickpeas, tomatoes and basil through the couscous. Season with salt and plenty of black pepper.

CHEFS NOTE
Don't worry if you haven't got any fresh basil, it's still worth making without it.

HERBED RICE & CHICKPEAS

315
calories per
serving

Ingredients

- 125g/4oz microwave rice
- 1 garlic clove
- ½ red onion
- 2 cherry tomatoes
- ½ tsp crushed chilli flakes
- 1 tsp grated ginger

- Large pinch of salt
- 1 tbsp lime juice
- ¼ cucumber
- Small bunch of fresh mint & coriander
- 75g/3oz tinned chickpeas, drained
- Salt & pepper to taste

Method

1 Get the rice cooked in the microwave. Check the packet instructions (it usually take about 1-2 minutes).

2 Meanwhile put all the other ingredients, except the chickpeas, in the food processor and give it a blast until everything is chopped up (don't turn it into a puree, just pulse a couple of times).

3 When the rice is ready tip into a bowl and fluff it up with a fork. Add everything from the food processor and combine really well, along with the chickpeas.

4 Check the seasoning and eat up!

CHEFS NOTE
This is a great make-ahead recipe for a work day lunch or on-the-go.

FLAGEOLET BEAN LUNCH BOX

360 calories per serving

Ingredients

- 1 garlic clove, crushed
- 1 tbsp wine or cider vinegar
- 1 tsp lemon juice
- ½ tsp crushed chilli flakes
- Large pinch of salt

- 200g/7oz tinned flageolet beans, drained
- 1 baby gem lettuce
- 75g/3oz tinned sweetcorn, drained
- 4 cherry tomatoes
- Salt & pepper to taste

Method

1 First you need to make your dressing so grab a bowl and mix up the garlic, vinegar, lemon, crushed chillies and salt (alter the balance to suit your own taste).

2 Give the flageolet beans a quick rinse in cold water, dry them off and add to the same bowl. Mix everything up and put to one side for a minute.

3 Shred the lettuce, halve the cherry tomatoes and get them set up in a shallow bowl. Tip the dressed flageolet beans over and pile the drained sweetcorn on top.

4 If you've got any fresh flat leaf parsley get that sprinkled over too, if not don't worry.

5 Load it into an airtight lunchbox and keep it in the fridge until lunchtime comes around.

CHEFS NOTE

Packed with good carbs there's no reason to miss out on a decent lunch on your fast days!

TURKEY BURGER

310 calories per serving

Ingredients

- 1 turkey breast weighting 125g/4oz
- 2 tsp teriyaki sauce
- 1 slice tinned pineapple
- 1 handful of shredded lettuce

- 1 regular soft wholemeal roll
- Low cal cooking oil spray
- Salt & pepper to taste

Method

1 Preheat the grill to medium/high heat.

2 Give the turkey breast a few bashes with a rolling pin to make it tender, season and brush with teriyaki sauce. Stick it under the grill with the pineapple ring at the side and cook for about 10 minutes or until it's cooked through (take the pineapple out sooner if it's cooking too fast).

3 When the turkey is ready pile it into the roll with the pineapple ring on top, add the lettuce and put the lid on. Open wide and eat!

CHEFS NOTE

Like it hot? Pile on some fresh chillies too.

TUNA, OLIVES & PEPPER LUNCH

395 calories per serving

Ingredients

- 1 tsp lemon juice
- 1 tsp olive oil
- 1 tsp balsamic vinegar
- 1 tsp Dijon mustard
- ½ garlic clove, crushed
- ½ red onion, sliced
- 1 pepper, deseeded & sliced
- 2 vine ripened tomatoes, sliced
- 75g/3oz rocket
- 125g/4oz tinned tuna, drained
- 6 pitted black olives, sliced
- Salt & pepper to taste

Method

1 Make a dressing by mixing up the lemon, oil, vinegar, mustard & garlic with a good pinch of salt.

2 Load the onions, peppers, sliced tomatoes & rocket in a shallow bowl and use a fork to flake the tuna over the top. Pour over the dressing and add the olives.

3 Season with lots of black pepper and eat up.

CHEFS NOTE

A quick and easy lunch packed with omega oils.

CHICKEN & PEA EGG FRIED 'RICE'

305 calories per serving

Ingredients

- 200g/7oz cauliflower florets
- 1 tsp olive oil
- ½ onion, chopped
- 1 garlic clove, crushed
- ½ red pepper, chopped & deseeded
- 1 tsp soy sauce
- 1 small free-range egg
- 50g/2oz peas
- 50g/2oz cooked chicken breast, shredded
- 2 spring onions/scallions, chopped
- Salt & pepper to taste

Method

1 Place the cauliflower florets in a food processor and pulse a few times until the cauliflower is the size of rice grains.

2 Place the 'rice' in a microwavable dish, cover and cook on full power for about 2 minutes or until it's piping hot. When it's done put to one side

3 Whilst the rice is cooking heat the oil in a frying pan and sauté the onion, garlic & peppers for a few minutes. Add the chicken and peas to the pan and cook for 2 minutes longer.

4 Add the 'rice' to the pan along with the soy sauce and move around well. Break the egg into the centre and quickly stir-fry until you see the egg 'set'.

5 Tip into a bowl and sprinkle the chopped spring onions over the top.

CHEFS NOTE

If you are using frozen peas, cook in boiling water for a couple of minutes first and then add to the rice.

STEAMED SALMON & BROCCOLI LUNCH BOWL

350 calories per serving

Ingredients

- 1 skinless salmon fillet weighing 150g/5oz
- 1 tbsp soy sauce
- 1 tbsp lime juice
- 200g/7oz tenderstem broccoli, roughly chopped

- 50g/2oz mangetout or sugarsnap peas
- ½ cucumber, diced
- ½ red pepper, deseeded & sliced
- 1 tbsp freshly chopped coriander/cilantro
- 1 tsp sesame seeds
- Salt & pepper to taste

Method

1 Season the salmon and brush with the soy sauce and lime juice. Place in the bottom tier of a steamer. Cover with the lid and leave to steam for 5 minutes.

2 Add the broccoli and mangetout to the second tier of the steamer, replace the lid and steam for another 4 minutes or until the fish is cooked through.

3 Take the veg out of the steamer and rinse under cold water for a second so that it stops cooking – you don't want it too soft.

4 Dry the veg off and tip into a bowl. Flake the salmon over the top. Add the cucumber, peppers and coriander. Sprinkle with sesame seeds and you are ready to go.

CHEFS NOTE

Sesame seeds are packed with calcium, magnesium & zinc.

SPICED KING PRAWN COUSCOUS

360 calories per serving

Ingredients

- 50g/2oz couscous
- 80ml/⅓ cup boiling hot chicken stock
- 1 red chilli
- 1 garlic clove
- 2 tsp lemon juice
- 1 tsp white wine vinegar
- ½ red onion
- Pinch of salt
- 150g/5oz cooked king prawns/jumbo shrimp
- 50g/2oz spinach
- Salt & pepper to taste

Method

1 Put the couscous & stock in a bowl, cover and leave for a couple of minutes whilst the couscous absorbs the stock.

2 Meanwhile add the chilli, garlic, lemon juice, vinegar, onion & salt to a food processor and whizz into a paste. Remove the blade, add the prawns and combine well with a spoon.

3 Use a fork to fluff up the couscous and combine with the spiced prawns. Pile on top of the spinach and eat.

CHEFS NOTE

Leaving the seeds in the chilli will make this nice and spicy.

MANFOOD

UNDER 500 CALORIES

FAST PRAWN STIR-FRY

420 calories per serving

Ingredients

- 50g/2oz mushrooms, sliced
- 1 garlic clove, crushed
- ½ onion, sliced
- 1 tsp grated ginger
- 60ml/¼ cup vegetable stock
- 125g/4oz raw king prawns/jumbo shrimp

- ½ tsp crushed chilli flakes
- 75g/3oz sugar snap peas
- 125g/4oz microwave rice
- Low cal cooking oil spray
- Salt & pepper to taste

Method

1 Throw the mushrooms, garlic, sliced onion & ginger in a frying pan with some low cal spray and gently sauté for a few minutes until things start to soften up (add a splash of water to the pan if you need to).

2 Turn up the heat, add the stock, prawns, crushed chillies & peas and continue cooking on medium heat for a couple of minutes.

3 Meanwhile cook the rice in the microwave. Check the packet instructions (it usually takes about 1-2 minutes).

4 Tip the cooked rice in the pan and continue stir-frying until the prawns are pink and cooked through & the stock has been absorbed.

5 Season and serve. Job done.

CHEFS NOTE
Have some herbs? Roughly chop some fresh coriander and spring onions for garnish.

CHICKEN SWEET CHILLI NOODLES

420 calories per serving

Ingredients

- 50g/2oz dried fine egg noodles
- ½ vegetable stock cube
- 100g/3½oz peas
- 1 tbsp sweet chilli sauce
- 1 tsp soy sauce
- 100g/3½oz cooked chicken breast, shredded
- 4 spring onions/scallions, chopped
- Lime wedges to serve
- Salt & pepper to taste

Method

1 Crumble the stock in a pan of boiling water and stir to dissolve. Add the egg noodles & peas, cover and leave to cook on the hob for a few minutes until the peas are cooked through and the noodles are tender.

2 Drain the noodles and mix with the sweet chilli and soy sauce. Get this set up in a bowl, place the shredded chicken on top (hot or cold) and sprinkle with the chopped spring onions.

3 Serve with lime wedges and, if you've got any, some chopped flat leaf parsley.

CHEFS NOTE
Sweet & sticky this can also be served cold as a handy lunchbox meal.

THAI CURRY & RICE

440 calories per serving

Ingredients

- 125g/4oz microwave rice
- 125g/4oz raw king prawns/jumbo shrimp
- ½ onion, chopped
- 2 tsp Thai green curry paste
- 120ml/½ cup low fat coconut milk
- 50g/2oz watercress
- Low cal cooking oil spray
- Salt & pepper to taste

Method

1 Get the rice cooked in the microwave. Check the packet instructions (it usually takes about 1-2 minutes).

2 Meanwhile throw the onions and prawns in a frying pan with some low cal spray and gently sauté for a couple of minutes (add a splash of water to the pan if you need to.)

3 Stir through the curry paste and coconut milk, cover and leave to cook for a few minutes until the prawns are pink and cooked thorough.

4 Tip the rice into a bowl. Pour over the curry and top with the watercress.

CHEFS NOTE
The watercress gives this simple curry a nice little crunch.

ZUCCHINI TAGLIATELLE

495
calories per
serving

Ingredients

- 75g/3oz tagliatelle
- 1 slice lean, back bacon
- 1 garlic clove, crushed
- 200g/7oz courgettes, finely sliced lengthways

- 1 medium free-range egg
- 60ml/¼ cup low fat cream
- 2 tsp grated Parmesan cheese
- Low cal cooking oil spray
- Salt & pepper to taste

Method

1 Put the pasta in a pan of salted boiling water. Cover and cook for about 10 minutes or until it's tender.

2 Meanwhile finely chop the bacon and throw it in a frying pan to gently cook along with the garlic & courgettes in a little low cal spray for about 5 minutes or until it's cooked through (add a dash of water to the pan if you need to).

3 Beat together the egg and cream in a cup. Drain the pasta, return to the pan and add the cooked veg. Pour over the egg and cream and combine really well on a gently heat (it'll only take about 10 seconds to get the job done).

4 Tip it into a shallow bowl, sprinkle the Parmesan over the top and eat up.

CHEFS NOTE
Don't mix the egg, cream and pasta on the heat for too long. You don't want it to end up looking like scrambled egg.

SKINNY SAUSAGE PENNE

SERVES 1

440 calories per serving

Ingredients

- 50g/2oz penne
- 125g/4oz venison sausage
- 1 garlic clove, crushed
- ½ onion, sliced
- 250ml/1 cup tomato passata/sauce
- ½ tsp each salt & brown sugar
- 1 tsp Worcesteshire sauce/A1 steak sauce
- 75g/3oz kale
- Low cal cooking oil spray
- Salt & pepper to taste

Method

1 Put the pasta in a pan of salted boiling water. Cover and cook for about 10 minutes or until it's tender.

2 Meanwhile get the sausages cooking in a frying pan with the garlic & sliced onions in a little low cal spray for about 8-10 minutes or until the sausages are cooked through (add a splash of water to the pan if you need to loosen up the onions).

3 While the sausage and pasta are cooking put together the sauce. This is simple: combine the passata, salt, sugar and Worcestershire sauce in a pan and gently cook on a low heat.

4 Just before the pasta is finished add the kale to the pasta pan and cook for 2 minutes. Drain the pasta & kale, return to the pan and add the tomato sauce. Slice the sausages into discs and throw these in too, along with the onions. Combine everything and dig in.

CHEFS NOTE
There's a lot going on in this recipe but every part is super easy…just keep an eye on your timings and it'll come together.

SQUASH & SAGE SPAGHETTI

430 calories per serving

Ingredients

- 150g/5oz butternut squash flesh, peeled & deseeded
- 75g/3oz spaghetti
- 2 tsp freshly chopped sage
- ½ onion, chopped
- 1 garlic clove, crushed

- 60ml/¼ cup hot vegetable stock
- 2 tbsp low fat cream
- 2 tsp grated Parmesan cheese
- Low cal cooking oil spray
- Salt & pepper to taste

Method

1 Finely chop the butternut squash. Put the pasta in a pan of salted boiling water, cover and cook for about 10 minutes or until it's tender.

2 Meanwhile gently sauté the squash, sage, onion & garlic in a little low cal spray for about 8-10 minutes or until it's softened and cooked through (add a dash of water to the pan if you need to loosen it up).

3 Drain the pasta. When the squash is ready throw it into a blender along with the hot stock. Give it a whizz until you have a smooth sauce and add a little more water or stock to alter the consistency if you need to.

4 Stir through the cream and tip it into the pan along with the drained pasta. Toss really well, get it plated up, sprinkle over the Parmesan and serve.

CHEFS NOTE

Use dried sage if you don't have any fresh to hand.

PEANUT & PRAWN NOODLE SALAD

405 calories per serving

Ingredients

- 50g/2oz dried fine egg noodles
- ½ vegetable stock cube
- 1 tbsp soy sauce
- 1 tbsp low fat peanut butter
- 2 tsp lime juice
- 4 cooked shelled king Prawns
- ¼ cucumber, finely chopped
- 4 spring onions/scallions, chopped
- Salt & pepper to taste

Method

1 Crumble the stock in a pan of boiling water and stir to dissolve. Add the egg noodles, cover and leave to cook on the hob for a few minutes until the noodles are tender.

2 Meanwhile make up the salad dressing by combining together the soy, peanut butter, & lime juice. When the noodles are ready toss the dressing through them.

3 Tip into a bowl and load over the chopped cucumber, king prawns and spring onions.

CHEFS NOTE
Season with plenty of soy sauce.

STEAK & CHIPS

440 calories per serving

Ingredients

- 150g/5oz sweet potatoes, cut into chips
- 150g/5oz trimmed sirloin or fillet steak
- 50g/2oz spinach
- 1 tbsp low fat cream
- Low cal cooking oil spray
- Salt & pepper to taste

Method

1 Preheat the oven to 200C/400F/Gas 6

2 Spray the 'chips' with a little low cal oil and season well with salt. Put these on a baking tray and place in the oven for 20 minutes.

3 Meanwhile season the steak and spray with a little low cal oil.

4 After the chips have been cooking for 20 minutes place a non-stick frying pan on a high heat and let it get smoking hot.

5 Add the steak to the pan and cook for 2 minutes each side (turning once). When it's done place it on a chopping board to 'rest' for a few minutes.

6 Throw the spinach into the steak pan with the cream, place on a low/medium heat and wilt for a minute or two. By the time you've done this the chips should be ready too.

7 Arrange everything on a plate and get stuck into the best steak and chips you are likely to find on a fast day.

CHEFS NOTE

Depending on the thickness of the steak two minutes each side should leave it fairly rare. Increase the cooking time if that doesn't suit you.

CHICKEN WITH A QUICK TOMATO SAUCE

405 calories per serving

Ingredients

- 1 skinless chicken breast weighing 150g/5oz
- 250ml/1 cup tomato passata/sauce
- 2 tbsp freshly chopped basil
- 1 tsp Worcestershire sauce
- 1 tbsp tomato puree/paste
- ½ tsp each salt & brown sugar
- 125g/4oz microwave rice
- Low cal cooking oil spray
- Salt & pepper to taste

Method

1 Preheat the grill to a medium/high heat.

2 Bash the chicken a few times with a rolling pin. Season, spray with a little low cal oil and cook under the grill for about 10-12 minutes or until the chicken is cooked through (turning a couple of times during cooking).

3 Meanwhile throw the passata, basil, Worcestershire sauce, puree, salt & sugar into a saucepan and cook over a gentle heat.

4 When the chicken is nearly ready get the rice cooked in the microwave. Check the packet instructions (it usually takes about 1-2 minutes).

5 Tip the rice into a bowl. Place the bashed grilled chicken on top and pour over the sauce. Easy.

CHEFS NOTE

This is a ridiculously easy tomato sauce to make for chicken & rice when you are in a rush.

MANFOOD

EXTRAS

CAULIFLOWER 'RICE'

50 calories per serving

Ingredients

- **1 large cauliflower head (approx. 800g/1¾lb)**

Method

1 Split the cauliflower head into florets and place in a food processor.

2 Whizz until the cauliflower is the size of rice grains.

3 Place the 'rice' in a microwavable dish, cover and cook on full power for about 4 minutes or until it's piping hot (cook for less time if you are only heating one portion).

---

50 calories per serving

COURGETTE SPAGHETTI

Ingredients

- **300g/11oz courgettes**

Method

1 Use the peeler to move along the side of the courgettes lengthwise to make long, flat slices. When you get close to the seed core, turn and begin slicing along another side. Continue until all you have left is a seedy core.

2 Discard the core and then cut the slices lengthwise using a knife to make the spaghetti. Simple and carb free.

HOMEMADE SALSA

50 calories per serving

Ingredients

- 125g/4oz fresh tomatoes, finely chopped
- ½ onion, finely chopped
- 1 green chilli, deseeded & finely chopped
- Small bunch fresh coriander/cilantro, finely chopped
- Salt, to taste
- Lime juice, to taste

Method

Combine all ingredients together and serve.

30 calories per serving

CUCUMBER SALAD SNACK

Ingredients

- ½ cucumber
- 2 tsp lemon juice
- Pinch of salt
- Pinch of brown sugar
- Pinch of dried crushed chillies
- 1 tsp fresh coriander/cilantro, chopped
- 1 tsp fresh mint, chopped

Method

1 Use the peeler to move along the side of the courgettes lengthwise to make long, flat slices. When you get close to the seed core, turn and begin slicing along another side. Continue until all you have left is a seedy core.

2 Discard the core and then cut the slices lengthwise using a knife to make the spaghetti. Simple and carb free.

SEA SALT SUGAR SNAP PEAS

65 calories per serving

Ingredients

- 75g/3oz sugar snap peas
- 1 tsp low fat 'butter' spread
- 1 tsp crushed sea salt
- 1 tsp chopped fresh mint or basil

Method

Place the peas in a pan of boiling water for 1 minute. Drain and then add the 'butter' and chopped herbs into pan. When the 'butter' has melted transfer to a bowl and sprinkle with sea salt.

75 calories per serving

CARROT & CELERY SALAD

Ingredients

- 1 carrot peeled & grated
- 1 tsp lemon juice
- 1 celery stalk, chopped
- 1 slice of tinned pineapple, chopped
- Pinch of salt

Method

Combine all ingredients well in a bowl and serve.

CONVERSION CHART: DRY INGREDIENTS

Metric	Imperial
7g	¼ oz
15g	½ oz
20g	¾ oz
25g	1 oz
40g	1½oz
50g	2oz
60g	2½oz
75g	3oz
100g	3½oz
125g	4oz
140g	4½oz
150g	5oz
165g	5½oz
175g	6oz
200g	7oz
225g	8oz
250g	9oz
275g	10oz
300g	11oz
350g	12oz
375g	13oz
400g	14oz

Metric	Imperial
425g	15oz
450g	1lb
500g	1lb 2oz
550g	1¼lb
600g	1lb 5oz
650g	1lb 7oz
675g	1½lb
700g	1lb 9oz
750g	1lb 11oz
800g	1¾lb
900g	2lb
1kg	2¼lb
1.1kg	2½lb
1.25kg	2¾lb
1.35kg	3lb
1.5kg	3lb 6oz
1.8kg	4lb
2kg	4½lb
2.25kg	5lb
2.5kg	5½lb
2.75kg	6lb

CONVERSION CHART: LIQUID MEASURES

Metric	Imperial	US
25ml	1fl oz	
60ml	2fl oz	¼ cup
75ml	2½ fl oz	
100ml	3½fl oz	
120ml	4fl oz	½ cup
150ml	5fl oz	
175ml	6fl oz	
200ml	7fl oz	
250ml	8½ fl oz	1 cup
300ml	10½ fl oz	
360ml	12½ fl oz	
400ml	14fl oz	
450ml	15½ fl oz	
600ml	1 pint	
750ml	1¼ pint	3 cups
1 litre	1½ pints	4 cups

Other
COOKNATION
TITLES

If you enjoyed '**MANFOOD: 5:2 Fast Diet Meals For Men**' we'd really appreciate your feedback. Reviews help others decide if this is the right book for them so a moment of your time would be appreciated.

Thank you.

You may also be interested in other titles in the CookNation series. Including the popular calorie counted 'Skinny' series.
You can find all the following great titles by searching under '**CookNation**'.

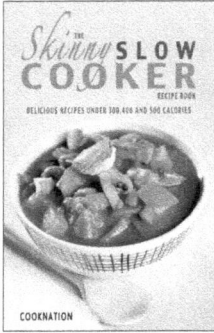

THE SKINNY SLOW COOKER RECIPE BOOK

Delicious Recipes Under 300, 400 And 500 Calories.

Paperback / eBook

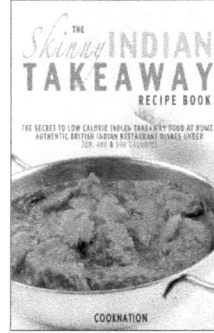

THE SKINNY INDIAN TAKEAWAY RECIPE BOOK

Authentic British Indian Restaurant Dishes Under 300, 400 And 500 Calories. The Secret To Low Calorie Indian Takeaway Food At Home.

Paperback / eBook

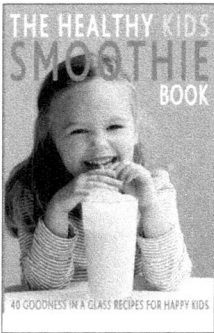

THE HEALTHY KIDS SMOOTHIE BOOK

40 Delicious Goodness In A Glass Recipes for Happy Kids.

eBook

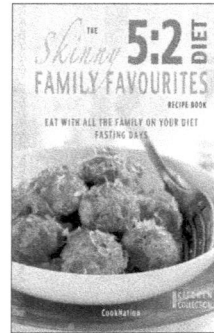

THE SKINNY 5:2 FAST DIET FAMILY FAVOURITES RECIPE BOOK

Eat With All The Family On Your Diet Fasting Days.

Paperback / eBook

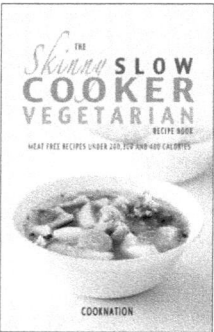

THE SKINNY SLOW COOKER VEGETARIAN RECIPE BOOK

40 Delicious Recipes Under 200, 300 And 400 Calories.

Paperback / eBook

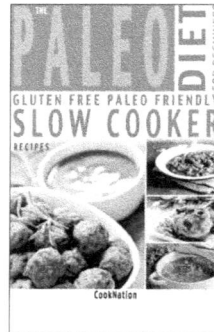

THE PALEO DIET FOR BEGINNERS SLOW COOKER RECIPE BOOK

Gluten Free, Everyday Essential Slow Cooker Paleo Recipes For Beginners.

eBook

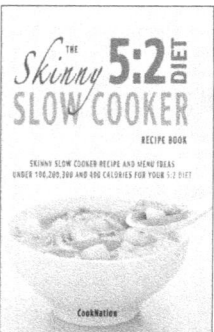

THE SKINNY 5:2 SLOW COOKER RECIPE BOOK

Skinny Slow Cooker Recipe And Menu Ideas Under 100, 200, 300 & 400 Calories For Your 5:2 Diet.

Paperback / eBook

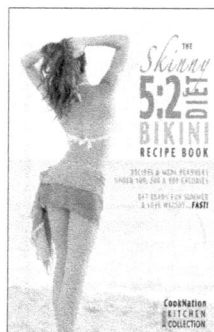

THE SKINNY 5:2 BIKINI DIET RECIPE BOOK

Recipes & Meal Planners Under 100, 200 & 300 Calories. Get Ready For Summer & Lose Weight...FAST!

Paperback / eBook

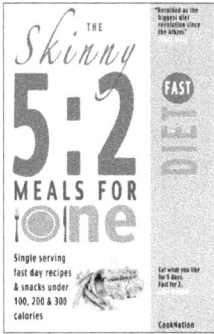

THE SKINNY 5:2 FAST DIET MEALS FOR ONE

Single Serving Fast Day Recipes & Snacks Under 100, 200 & 300 Calories.

Paperback / eBook

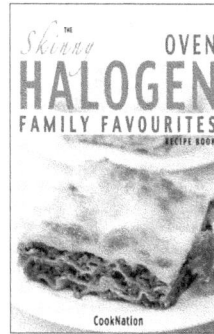

THE SKINNY HALOGEN OVEN FAMILY FAVOURITES RECIPE BOOK

Healthy, Low Calorie Family Meal-Time Halogen Oven Recipes Under 300, 400 and 500 Calories.

Paperback / eBook

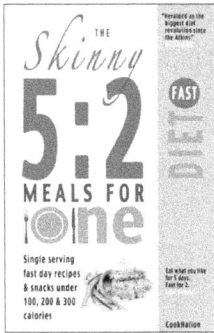

THE SKINNY 5:2 FAST DIET VEGETARIAN MEALS FOR ONE

Single Serving Fast Day Recipes & Snacks Under 100, 200 & 300 Calories.

Paperback / eBook

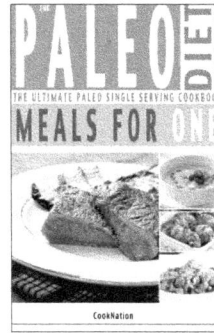

THE PALEO DIET FOR BEGINNERS MEALS FOR ONE

The Ultimate Paleo Single Serving Cookbook.

Paperback / eBook

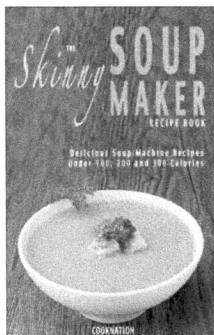

THE SKINNY SOUP MAKER RECIPE BOOK

Delicious Low Calorie, Healthy and Simple Soup Recipes Under 100, 200 and 300 Calories. Perfect For Any Diet and Weight Loss Plan.

Paperback / eBook

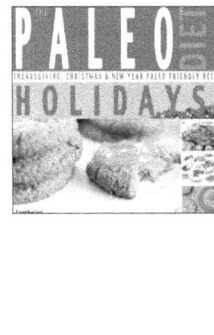

THE PALEO DIET FOR BEGINNERS HOLIDAYS

Thanksgiving, Christmas & New Year Paleo Friendly Recipes.
eBook

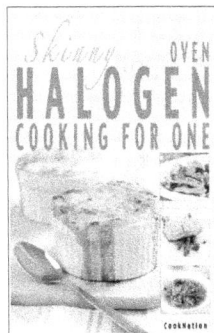

SKINNY HALOGEN OVEN COOKING FOR ONE

Single Serving, Healthy, Low Calorie Halogen Oven RecipesUnder 200, 300 and 400 Calories.

Paperback / eBook

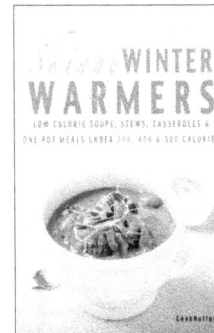

SKINNY WINTER WARMERS RECIPE BOOK

Soups, Stews, Casseroles & One Pot Meals Under 300, 400 & 500 Calories.

Paperback / eBook

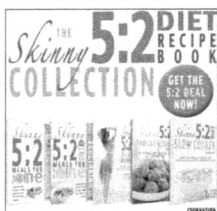

THE SKINNY 5:2 DIET RECIPE BOOK COLLECTION

All The 5:2 Fast Diet Recipes You'll Ever Need. All Under 100, 200, 300, 400 And 500 Calories.

eBook

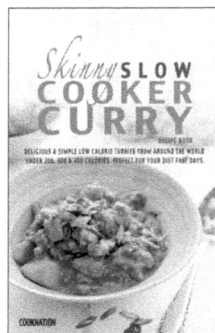

THE SKINNY SLOW COOKER CURRY RECIPE BOOK

Low Calorie Curries From Around The World.

Paperback / eBook

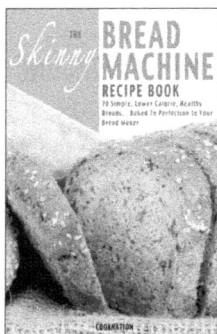

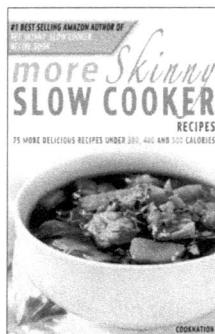

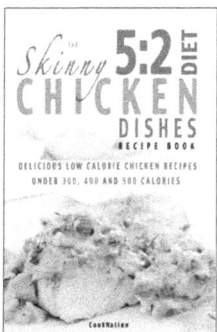

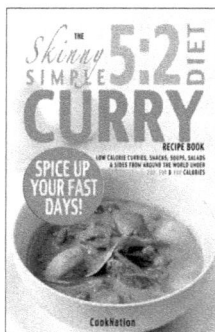

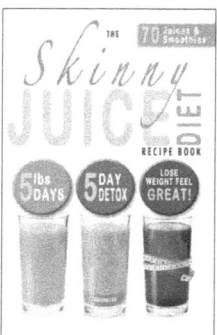

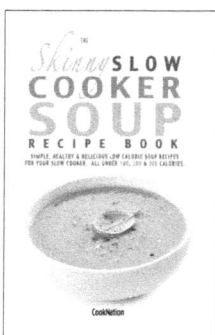

THE SKINNY BREAD MACHINE RECIPE BOOK

70 Simple, Lower Calorie, Healthy Breads...Baked To Perfection In Your Bread Maker.

Paperback / eBook

MORE SKINNY SLOW COOKER RECIPES

75 More Delicious Recipes Under 300, 400 & 500 Calories.

Paperback / eBook

THE SKINNY 5:2 DIET CHICKEN DISHES RECIPE BOOK

Delicious Low Calorie Chicken Dishes Under 300, 400 & 500 Calories.

Paperback / eBook

THE SKINNY 5:2 CURRY RECIPE BOOK

Spice Up Your Fast Days With Simple Low Calorie Curries, Snacks, Soups, Salads & Sides Under 200, 300 & 400 Calories.

Paperback / eBook

THE SKINNY JUICE DIET RECIPE BOOK

5lbs, 5 Days. The Ultimate Kick- Start Diet and Detox Plan to Lose Weight & Feel Great!

Paperback / eBook

THE SKINNY SLOW COOKER SOUP RECIPE BOOK

Simple, Healthy & Delicious Low Calorie Soup Recipes For Your Slow Cooker. All Under 100, 200 & 300 Calories.

Paperback / eBook

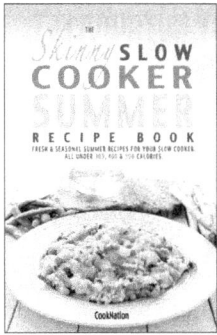

THE SKINNY SLOW COOKER SUMMER RECIPE BOOK

Fresh & Seasonal Summer Recipes For Your Slow Cooker. All Under 300, 400 And 500 Calories.

Paperback / eBook

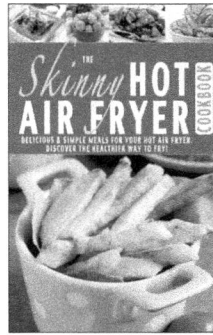

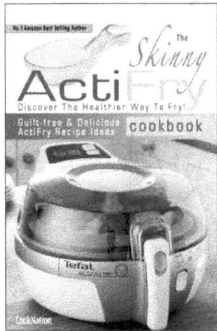

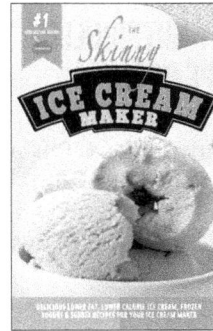

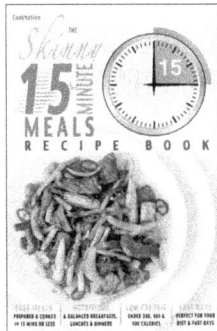

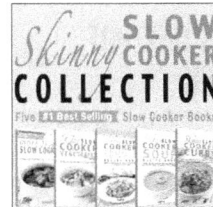

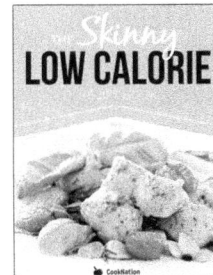

THE SKINNY HOT AIR FRYER COOKBOOK

Delicious & Simple Meals For Your Hot Air Fryer: Discover The Healthier Way To Fry.

Paperback / eBook

THE SKINNY ACTIFRY COOKBOOK

Guilt-free and Delicious ActiFry Recipe Ideas: Discover The Healthier Way to Fry!

Paperback / eBook

THE SKINNY ICE CREAM MAKER

Delicious Lower Fat, Lower Calorie Ice Cream, Frozen Yogurt & Sorbet Recipes For Your Ice Cream Maker.

Paperback / eBook

THE SKINNY 15 MINUTE MEALS RECIPE BOOK

Delicious, Nutritious & Super-Fast Meals in 15 Minutes Or Less. All Under 300, 400 & 500 Calories.

Paperback / eBook

THE SKINNY SLOW COOKER COLLECTION

5 Fantastic Books of Delicious, Diet-friendly Skinny Slow Cooker Recipes: ALL Under 200, 300, 400 & 500 Calories!
eBook

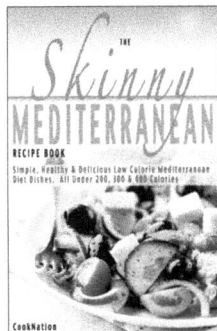

THE SKINNY MEDITERRANEAN RECIPE BOOK

Simple, Healthy & Delicious Low Calorie Mediterranean Diet Dishes. All Under 200, 300 & 400 Calories.

Paperback / eBook

THE SKINNY LOW CALORIE RECIPE BOOK

Great Tasting, Simple & Healthy Meals Under 300, 400 & 500 Calories. Perfect For Any Calorie Controlled Diet.

Paperback / eBook

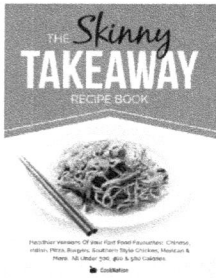

THE SKINNY TAKEAWAY RECIPE BOOK

Healthier Versions Of Your Fast Food Favourites: All Under 300, 400 & 500 Calories.

Paperback / eBook

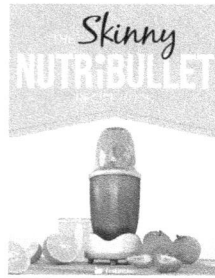

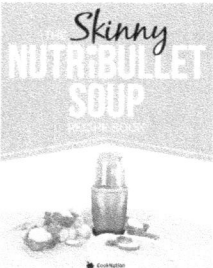

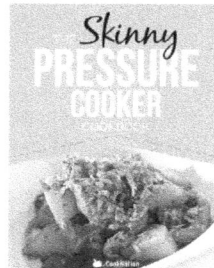

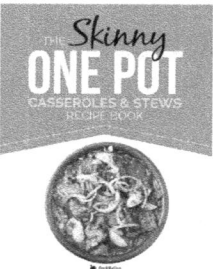

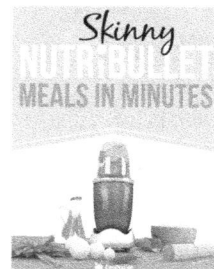

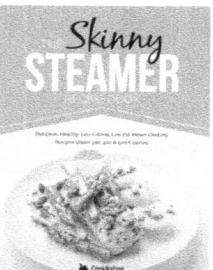

THE SKINNY NUTRIBULLET RECIPE BOOK

80+ Delicious & Nutritious Healthy Smoothie Recipes. Burn Fat, Lose Weight and Feel Great!

Paperback / eBook

THE SKINNY NUTRIBULLET SOUP RECIPE BOOK

Delicious, Quick & Easy, Single Serving Soups & Pasta Sauces For Your Nutribullet. All Under 100, 200, 300 & 400 Calories!

Paperback / eBook

THE SKINNY PRESSURE COOKER COOKBOOK

USA ONLY
Low Calorie, Healthy & Delicious Meals, Sides & Desserts. All Under 300, 400 & 500 Calories.

Paperback / eBook

THE SKINNY ONE-POT RECIPE BOOK

Simple & Delicious, One-Pot Meals. All Under 300, 400 & 500 Calories

Paperback / eBook

THE SKINNY NUTRIBULLET MEALS IN MINUTES RECIPE BOOK

Quick & Easy, Single Serving Suppers, Snacks, Sauces, Salad Dressings & More Using Your Nutribullet. All Under 300, 400 & 500 Calories

Paperback / eBook

THE SKINNY STEAMER RECIPE BOOK

Healthy, Low Calorie, Low Fat Steam Cooking Recipes Under 300, 400 & 500 Calories.

Paperback / eBook